Healthy Beauty, Ageless Beauty

Denie Hiestand

ISBN-13: 978-1537321844
ISBN-10: 1537321846

DEDICATION

I dedicate this book to all my clients I have seen over the years who have helped push my understanding on *how* this body works and what causes it to malfunction. Now I can share my knowledge with you, so we can all help make this human experience more healthy and beautiful.

CONTENTS

ACKNOWLEDGMENTS

We all live a busy life, and it is a big commitment to take the time to put pen to paper. So thank you Shala, Narah, and Shelley. You put the right amount of pressure on me to just do it.

Also, from the bottom of my heart, I thank my long-time friend and favorite Oregonian, Anna Kyle Skidgel. You took my outpouring and turned it into something readable without taking *me* out of the words. I am so honored and blessed by your commitment to this project and for your editing skills.

And thank you EiffelMedia.com for the cover design.

Healthy Beauty, Ageless Beauty

Foreword

By Dame Adrienne Papp

The brilliance of Denie Hiestand is obvious from his words as he describes the electrical nature of *how* our body works, and in general, the human existence.

After reading this well-written summary of how we are "wired," I now have the clearest understanding about the most basic principals that we scientifically know from quantum physics, but are shy to apply in our daily lives. Hiestand gets practical and injects a great sense of humor, which makes this book not only fun to read, but also a must-read. I do not promise that your life will change, I KNOW it will.

Hiestand takes a refreshingly, unapologetic approach to challenge commonly accepted views on health and beauty. By masterfully describing *how* the body works, Hiestand's down-to-earth, logical explanations make seemingly complex concepts accessible and understandable so that no confusion remains.

In order for us to feel vibrant and ready to create positive changes in our lives and in the world, we must take time for renewal on a molecular level. Grant yourself the permission to step away from the "busyness" of your life, for physical and spiritual self-care, by absorbing and embodying these words. I invite you to let go of all that has come before this moment.

Surrender your entire being completely to the blessed

peace of understanding that you have all the power within you to create anything in your life, including healthy, ageless beauty.

Hiestand is a gift to the world; he offers you the choice to turn your attention away from darkness toward the light of divine life within. He moves you from fear into freedom and a higher consciousness for you to grow into who you TRULY are, and find your unlimited potential for *Healthy Beauty, Ageless Beauty*.

Dame Adrienne Papp

1. ENERGY IS EVERYTHING

There are millions of words written about health and beauty, and more millions written about those crazy terms: "anti-aging" and "ageless."

So yes; I hear you saying: "What? Another book on health, beauty, and anti-aging?"

Yea, I get it, and I react the same when I see yet another new book on these subjects. And if I read them I am usually, like you, confused, conflicted, and left with no real answers -- well not the answers I wanted at any rate.

Okay, so why another book on these subjects? Why would I take the time to put pen to paper (Well, tap keys on my computer at any rate.)? Maybe I am just like you; maybe I want to know not only *what* happens to this body of mine, but also *how* it happens and *how* to stop it happening.

The *what* that happens is easy: Hit finger with hammer,

big owie, pain and swelling, and with time all is well again. That's *what* happened. But *how* did the pain happen? *How* did the body repair itself? *How* did my brain know that some part of my body was injured? *How* did the cells respond; *how* did it all work? That's where *my* brain goes.

I remember as a young boy asking incessant questions every time my dad asked or told me to do something on the farm. My never-ending questions drove him nuts. I could always see *what* he wanted, but I always asked "Why?" and "How would this or that be the right thing to do or the right way to do it?" I think I left home at 17 to save my dad from an early grave -- bless his soul. I had the same issue with most of my school teachers: I just drove them to despair. Especially my science teacher, but not my engineering teacher: *That* I got. I not only understood the *what* happened, I understood the *how* it happened.

I loved engineering with a passion, because it's all about the *how*: how to build a bridge, how to design and build a sky scraper, how to build an airplane. Speaking of airplanes: One of the first jet airliners, the *Comet 4,* kept falling out of the sky and nobody knew why. The *what* happened was easy: the bloody thing broke and fell out of the sky. That's *what* happened. But the *why* and *how* were the tricky parts that took many months to figure out. You see, the main structural parts were solid metal and could take many more tons of stress than it took to hold the aircraft together in flight. But they broke.

The engineering guys and girls, and many scientists, had

to drill deep into something they had not dealt with before. You see, the chemistry of the metal was okay, but something else made the metal parts just break in half. Well it soon transpired that, as the aircraft traveled through the air, a resonance built up -- a vibration, an *electrical* field was generated (energy if you like) and that resonance -- that vibration -- was such that it affected the bonding of the atoms within the metal. The metal molecules got to a certain frequency, a certain energy vibration, and they just let go hands and the metal fell apart. It's what we now know as *metal fatigue*. The electrical fields in the molecules got out of phase, and the energy bonding of the atoms failed, and the part broke, and down went the aircraft. We would not have modern reliable aircraft, tall buildings, and large bridges if the engineers did not look into and come to understand the *energy*, or electrical or vibrational side, of what takes place on a molecular level. The modern design process of all large structures and aircraft relies on this knowledge and understanding of energy. Because *all* things in this universe, *including* this *body* of ours are constructed and work on this *energy* reality. We are made of atoms. We are electrical. *We are energy*. And without understanding the *energy* part of life, we can never understand this body or this life we are living.

One more example: Years ago when our family was on the farm in New Zealand, I used to take in old, emotionally and physically broken race horses for my daughter, Karen, to ride. We used to let them loose in a large field so they could just be horses again, and Karen would love them and ride them. Anyhow, one old silver horse, Sam, was getting a bit ornery, and Karen didn't always finish her ride in the saddle. So it came to that time, as Sam was in pain and slept most of the day, to send him off to the large grassy field in the sky. When the vet was on the farm one day, I suggested we had better send Sam off, because I did not want him to suffer any longer.

So I went up to Sam and cradled his head in my arms as he lay there, giving him as much love as I could, while the vet went back to his rump, tapped it a couple of times and injected the bye-bye drug into his muscle. As the vet pushed in the syringe, Sam's head just let go into my arms and he passed.

"Hey," I said to the vet. "That's a drug you are using, right?"

"Yap, why?" he asked.

"How long does it take the blood to get pumped around a horse's body?" I asked.

He replied: "About three minutes or so."

Then I stepped back from the now-very-dead Sam and said: "Well, that could not have been a chemical reaction because as you were still pushing in the syringe, Sam's brain died and he was gone. The drug did not even get anywhere near his brain or heart or anywhere in that fraction of a second, so it can't be a chemical reaction. It must have been an *electrical action*, an electrical energy impulse process that turned off all the systems."

The vet stepped back, looked at me, looked at the horse, back at me and said: "You have just destroyed my 30 years of pharmaceutical knowledge. You are right: that could not have been a drug-only response."

That little episode started a long friendship between us, and we spent many hours discussing *how* life works on an electrical-impulse level or, as I say, as an energy system. We are energy and when the *energy* system goes wrong, disease and physical issues transpire.

So good people, this is why I am writing this little book. We all get told *what* is happening to our bodies. The *what* might be a heart attack, cancer, a bladder infection, or whatever, but we *never* get told the *how*, and without knowing the *how* we can never stop our diseases or even avoid them. Just like the engineers with the metal fatigue on those early jet aircraft, it was only by understanding *how* the metal broke in the first place that they are now able to prevent it from happening.

It's the same with our diseases, health, wellness, beauty and the aging process. Unless we understand the *how*, we will never stop our problems from happening. We need to understand the *energy* -- the electrical part of this body -- to get anywhere.

We came to live this life full of love, joy, and happiness, with vibrant health, and to look and feel great well into our old age. We came to dance, to be a little crazy, and to live every moment to its fullest. We cannot do that if we are ill, and we can't stop being ill unless we understand *how* this thing called a body works. We can't stop, cure, or change a darn thing unless we understand *how* it happens in the first place.

2. AN HONORABLE CAUSE

Most of us think that being honorable means doing the right thing for others, and that's true. But the most honorable action is being true to ourselves, honoring this body we live in, honoring our being-ness, our life, our being alive. Yes, we only really have our bodies in which to experience this life. Everybody and everything else is outside of us – add-ons, accompaniments. Sure those all make life way more meaningful for us, but they are only extensions of our own experiences. All our loves, joys, sorrows, fun and laughter, everybody and everything we experience outside of ourselves can only be experienced because we are *we*, us, living in this body of ours. Without this body that is *us*, we have no experience on this earth. Well, not that we remember anyhow.

And what is one of the most important things to all of us? To feel that we look good -- to feel we are beautiful. Really, it's true. How many of you look back at yourselves in the mirror each morning and wish you looked better -- hair better, eyes not so squinty, skin smoother, and damn those wrinkles, or whatever? Isn't all that self-criticism just a way of saying to ourselves we want to look good? Sure it is; and that's okay. In fact it's perfect. It's the way it should be. We all want that *youthful* and *ageless* thing going on. It's natural. All creatures experience it. It's in our genetic makeup to feel that we look good.

Look at how animals and birds preen themselves and each other. And it's not only to keep themselves and others clean; it really is so that they *feel* that they look good. My schizo cat just loves for me to rub her back hard, up and down. I love to finish with an up stroke to leave her coat all mucked up and going the wrong way just to see her reaction. She shakes herself, and then licks herself until all the hair is put back right and neat. Then the little prima donna, looks into the mirror -- really looks at herself -- and if one hair on her head is out of place, she will use her paw and gently make it right. She will look at herself over and over and do slight adjustments to her coat until she is happy with the way she looks. True story. Then she will just sit there, two inches away from the mirror, looking at herself, and purr. That cat!

So you see ladies, you haven't got this '*have to look good*' thing all to yourselves.

However, that youthful, anti-aging and beauty desire goes much deeper into our genetic makeup. When we strip away all our outer levels of consciousness, belief structures, and social patterning, that need to feel beautiful is completely related to finding a mate and breeding. Yes, really. The core of our wanting to feel beautiful is all to do with sex. And it has to be. That is the base genetic code that drives all living creatures. Without it, no species would survive. However, we mere males have it a bit less complicated when it comes to the genetically-coded breeding thing. We just want to be the biggest, strongest, bravest, loudest male in the herd. Damn civilization: It's taken half the fun out of being a man. Now we have to be all genteel like, sophisticated, gentlemanly, suave and debonair. Oh for the good old days when we boys snuck into the other tribe, grabbed the hot young things by the hair, and dragged them back to our camp. Real men we was. JUST KIDDING! I know, I know. Can't help myself sometimes. LOL.

But really, think about our genetic coding. Even today, young girls are attracted to the bad boy, the leader of the pack and all that. Ever seen young girls at a rock concert? Their behavior is that genetic coding thing working perfectly. They all want sex with the lead singer -- every one of them. The breeding urge is still so strong in all of us, and the survival of the fittest is still a significant part of our genetics, so it's natural that some girls will be drawn to the biggest, strongest, bravest, loudest boy. Totally natural and normal. But as parents, we hate it when our daughters act upon their deep, natural instincts and go for the boy from the wrong side of the tracks. Oh well, get over it, Dad! At least you know that her body is healthy enough to be in touch with her genetic coding. And hey, who are we to judge? It might just be the perfect match.

Okay, now we know that wanting to feel beautiful, and the desire to spend copious amounts of money on the latest anti-aging discoveries, trying to live the perfect anti-aging lifestyle, and using all the anti-aging strategies we can, is not *vanity* after all. It really is the most natural and, arguably, the most powerful genetically-coded behavior we can express. The urge to feel *youthful* and *ageless* and thus *beautiful*, is our base make up; therefore, let's own it, and most of all, *honor* it -- all of it -- and ourselves. Because we are all truly worth it. Wanting to feel beautiful is *An Honorable Cause*.

Now that we understand the *why* of wanting to be beautiful, youthful, and ageless, we had better understand the *how* in order to achieve what is a most natural desire.

3. ANTI-AGING LIFESTYLE

We all want it (anti-aging that is). We do all the anti-aging research; study up on the latest youthful, ageless breakthroughs; read the newest and latest anti-aging research and the latest anti-aging science; work on our anti-aging routines; seek out anti-aging therapies; and eat what we think are anti-aging foods. We look for the best anti-aging ingredients in the products we buy, try to use the best anti-aging creams and lotions on our skin, and try to live an anti-aging lifestyle. But really, are we getting anywhere? Are we getting value for our time and money? Are we achieving the anti-aging breakthroughs we are so desperately seeking? Do we look youthful and healthy enough?

Sadly, I think not.

So where did we go wrong? What part of this story did we miss? What part of this youthful anti-aging thing escaped us?

"Is it all BS., and have we wasted our money or what?" you ask.

Well, not really. Not entirely are you out of pocket; you have given yourselves a lot of information. However, most of it is fractured. You got a bit here, and a bit there. You went to this seminar and that seminar, listened to this person and that person, read a lot of books, got advice from this and that therapist, took a multitude of this herb and that drug or anti-aging potion, and still nothing, or very little, happened. Yes, I know the drill. Been there, done that, and ended up as confused and unhappy with the outcome as you are. Darn, tell me about it already.

Okay, enough of identifying the problem. You know the *what* only too well. You are living the *what* each and every day. You know *what* happened to your body, your life, your joy of living. So let's look at the *how*, because only when you understand *how* it happened, *how* you came to be in this miserable, painful, and maybe unhappy and dissatisfied place, can you even start to fix it. Recall the aircraft story. If we cannot understand the *how* some issue or problem happened, we can never change the outcome. Only by understanding *how* it happened, can we find solutions so it can't happen again. And if you do that, you get your body back, your life back. Simple, eh? Not. But highly possible. That's a big Hell Yes! But you have to learn some basic things about *how* your body works and then *you* have to *do it* -- right.

Right, now: If you don't want to learn some basic facts about your body -- stuff you have never been told about before -- and if you don't want to take responsibility for your body, just give this book to somebody else, or if you got the eBook version, just delete it from your computer or whatever, now. And go away and be miserable. . . . I used to say, "Go away and die," - but my Marketing Director (see Narah, I am trying) told me I can't say that, as it is too harsh and could upset some people. Okay sorry, I should be nice to you miserable lot, oops, you, wonderful people! You have paid me for this. Thank you. Groceries for a day. Yaaaaa, food! Well, maybe chocolate.

But before I go into the details of the *how* to fix this body we live in, I have an amazing story to tell you about a little old lady from Ashburton, a small rural town in the South Island of New Zealand. This story is about taking responsibility for one's body.

I had a small office that I worked out of as a Natural Health Consultant – well, really, it was an energy healing practice, calling myself a "Natural Health Consultant" got around all the licensing issues. I was regarded as the local witch doctor. Anyhow June (that's her name) was in her early 80s, overweight, toxic, riddled with arthritis, in chronic pain, and could only walk – barely -- with two sticks or a wheeled walker.

Her doctor had her on about five or six different medications, and as she was not getting any better, he suggested that she come see me. Yes, the town doctor sent me quite a few clients; he always said that he had no idea what I did, and did not want to know, but it seemed to work.

Anyhow, in comes June, almost bent over double, huffing and panting and hardly able to get one stick in front of herself to take the next shaky step. I remember that I had to lower my clinic table down to the bottom setting just so she could get onto it. After getting June as comfortable as I could, I started with my usual energy scan of her electromagnetic field.

Okay, a short side story to explain what I mean about scanning electromagnetic fields. I came into this world a rather strange wee lad. My interface with the world happened to be very different from most folks. From a very small child I could see the energy fields around objects and people. To me, the world *was* energy fields. I remember the time when my mum was going to send us kids (I was number five of seven) down to the neighbor's place to play with their kids. Well I kicked up a fuss, cried, and said I was not going. When mum asked why I did not want to go, I said: "They are all black and sad." You see, to me, the mother's energy (the field around her body) looked dark and distorted, almost scary in a way (she was a very unhappy, emotionally stressed lady), and most of the kids were not much better. I did not want to go anywhere near them. Of course, my mum told me not to be stupid, as there was no such thing as black, sad energy. But to me, what I could see was real.

However, I soon learned to shut my mouth about my world. I remember another time, when my sister ridiculed me in front of the whole family by telling them how she found me down the end of the farm in my secret hut, talking to the fairies. Yuh, my childhood was not the happiest, because nobody understood my world. So I shut down. For years.

Moving forward to my adult life, all this awareness came rushing back into my reality, in my late thirties, when I hit rock bottom. That's when my world went upside down, and I had to accept that my interface with the rest of the world was somewhat different than most. I had this strange ability to *see*, not only the electro-magnetic field around a body but, with my crazy-intense focus, every cell and its field *inside* the body as well. That's when I decided to study as many natural health modalities as I could in order to get my head around this thing that was my world.

To cut a long story short, I started to help my farmer friends with their pain and other health issues, as I could see what was going on in their bodies. I also experienced this strange energy phenomenon every time I went near, or put my hand on, a client: My body would generate tremendous heat (energy) and I could direct that energy through my hands into their cells and get them working again. So that's how I started to become well-known and ended up being flown all over the world for the last 30 years or so, putting bodies back together that others could not. My journey from farm boy to internationally recognized energy healer (and I don't like that word, as the cells do their own "healing." I just charge them up so they can work again), is outlined in my book, *Journey to Truth*. This book was the basis of the award-winning documentary, *One Man's Journey to Truth*, produced by Chesapeake Films.

So back to June. When done scanning her outer field, I looked at her and said: "Geez June, there is not much of you left."

She opened her eyes and replied in a very small voice: "Oh Denie, I can feel the life going out of me more each day. I feel like I am already dead."

I had started to scan again to find the most-stressed organ. "Darn," I thought to myself. "This lady is on her way out, nothing is working right, and all her organs are about to give up."

However, I could not find any real damage to any part of her system; she was just toxic and loaded with emotional trauma. She was basically dying of sadness. Sure her joints were real bad, and her pain was bad, but that was not killing her. It was just that her internal organs could not deal with the emotional loading anymore and were throwing in the towel.

I spent about an hour recharging her system to buy her some time, as I sorted out the best way forward. June got off my table feeling a million dollars -- so much more alive. She was so overjoyed and she could almost straighten her body.

Next I sat her down, went into her emotional body and cleared out some of the emotional energy (since the body's energy system is connected, it is one continuous field or circuit if you like, flowing through and around the body, it is quite easy for me to perceive what is emotional energy and then clean that energy out of a person's field), and then got her to talk to me about her life. Long story, but the guts of it were that her husband had died the year before, one of her daughters and her grandkids had moved to Australia, and she was all alone and felt her life was useless. She was the type of mother who lived for her husband and family. Never once could she remember doing something special for herself. She had lived outside of herself for over 50 years, never once really being in touch with her feelings; everybody else came first. And now she had nobody; she was dying.

Anyhow, I sent her on her way, feeling a whole lot better, with an appointment to come back the next week. That way I could see how her energy system was holding up. As I had brought the electrical charge up, I would then see if it was still running more energy than at the start of the first treatment. This would mean that I was right, and that in fact there was no, or very little, degeneration of the life-support organs. If there was some organ failure, her charge would be way down again. It's the same scenario with a flat car battery: Charge it up and put a load test on it, and you will see the condition of the battery. If it goes down really quickly, then the battery is on its way out; if the current stays for long enough, you know the battery is good. We are dealing with energy systems here, and all energy works on the same laws in the universe.

Well, by the time June was back in my office, I had figured out what to advise her regarding her recovery. You see, once I have been into somebody's energy field, I can bring the energy construct back to my consciousness and look at every cell to see the *how* and the *why* the system is not working. It's a bit like how a computer works: Only a very small amount of information is on the screen; 99.9% of the information is in the storage chips as an electrical impulse. If you know what file you want and know where it is, then a simple click, click, and that information is back on your screen as words. Well, the same with our consciousness: Once I have downloaded somebody's energy field, really their hard drive, or a part of it (don't need it all - way too much information that I don't need), I can bring it back to my screen -- my consciousness -- and see the information in my brain. It's all just energy impulses, and the energy fields hold all the information. It's how the universe works. It's how energy works. It's how your computer works; it's how our TVs work. It's how our brain works. It's how our body -- every last cell, every atom -- works. All the information is in the energy or electrical fields as impulses. Unfortunately, we are never taught this, so most of us have no idea that this is possible. By the way, it's also how I make my natural colostrum skin cream (*theCream*) work so darn well. I look at every electrical field.

So, June arrives on her next appointment date, and I sit her down and find her charge is still really good, so I was right, no real issues going on with her organs and she is feeling soooo much better. She thinks I am a magic man. Little does she know what's coming. I had written out instructions for her for the next six months: diet, movement, etc., but there was one issue that I knew she would not like. I asked her if she had ever looked at herself in the mirror, I mean not to do her hair and things like that, but really *looked at herself* -- the lady that was called June -- and really seen her.

"No," she said, "never done that."

Then I asked her if she had ever stood in front of a full-length mirror with no clothes on and looked at her body. I knew what was coming, so I just paused. Well, the poor old dear nearly had a heart attack.

She went red in the face, then white as a ghost with shock: "Oh my goodness," she said. "I would never do that."

"Bingo," I thought. "Hit the bulls-eye. Nailed her emotional block in under a minute."

You see, June had always lived for others. She had no concept herself -- of who or what *she* was. She had stuffed all her emotions until her cells could not deal with the energy loading. As the energy in the overloaded cell dropped, on went the pain receptors. That's all pain is: an electrical alarm signifying a low energy level in the cells. Her body was not even a thing to her, she lived outside of it. Well, now she had to turn around and walk back into herself and learn to love that which was her. She needed to honor and love *June*. If she could do that, all the pent-up emotional energy would just fall away, the cells would recharge, and all her pain would be gone. That is, as long as we could get the joints to rebuild, but I knew how to do that. Arthritis is so easy to reverse.

"Okay, Girl," I said to her. "This is your program.

Follow the diet outline to the letter (more on that in the 'anti-aging food' chapter), and this is your walk schedule, and this is for you to do at home: You are to look at yourself in your full-length mirror with no clothes on each day. You are to start by only looking at your feet. When you can love and really see your feet, move up. You are to do this each day until you can look at your whole body and smile and *feel* your own love."

Well the poor lady was beside herself; she just sat there crying. Remember, this was an old lady who could barely walk, needed help to go to the bathroom, could not even wash herself, wash dishes, or clean house. And here I was giving her unmentionable tasks to do, including walking each day.

I leaned down close to her and said, "June, do you want to live?"

"Yes, yes I do," she sobbed.

"Do you want your body back?" I asked.

"Yes, yes I do," she answered.

"Right," I said. "Just do what I say to the letter, or go away and die. It's one or the other. You choose. You have only one shot at this; it's now or your family buries you."

You should have seen the look on her face: total shock and dismay. I just kept my eyes on her and waited, just drilling my energy into her being.

She finally got control of herself and in a small voice said: "Okay, I will do it."

I said, "louder."

She said it again, and this time with some power in her voice. I leaned forward and wrapped my arms around her in a big bear hug. Then I told her that this would be the hardest thing she would ever do in her life, but in order to have a life, she must to do it. She nodded and said she understood.

Then I said to her, "If you don't do it all, and do it as I said, I will kick your saggy old ass."

Well that did it; she just roared with laughter and said: "Yes, it is a saggy old ass isn't it?" Then, "I want my body back. I want to feel alive again. I want to work in my garden again, and I want to see my grandkids."

Well, I did not see her again for some months, as I had to go to the States for three months of healing work and missed her on my return, because I was all over the country working. But about nine months after that session, I was in Ashburton, and from across the street came a voice:

"Denie, Denie!"

I looked around and this old lady was *running* across the road, skirt waving in the breeze and arms going in all directions.

"Oh my God," I said to myself. "It's June."

She hit me with such force she nearly knocked me over as her arms went around me in the biggest, most heartfelt hug I have ever had.

"Oh my God," I said to her. "Look at you. Damn, Girl, you look 30 years younger. My God, look at your skin, and where has that saggy old ass gone?"

Well we both nearly fell over laughing at that point. We then went to a coffee shop and sat for about an hour while June told me all about her last nine months. She did her walk every day as instructed, and had continued doing it. She started by going to the first power pole from her house, and each week she went to the next power pole, just like I told her to. She never deviated from the diet I gave her, not for one day.

But the most amazing thing she said to me was, "You know, Denie, it was those two things you said to me that got me through the worst pain, when I was about to give up, when I thought I could not take another step in the cold and rainy weather. It was when you told me: 'Do this and do it as I said to do it, or go away and die.' Every time I thought I could not go out of the house in the cold winter morning, I would hear your voice: '*Do it or go away and die.*' And I went out into the cold weather. The other thing was when I was walking and the pain was soooo bad and I would stop, unable to take another step, and your voice would come to me as if you were right beside me, clear as a bell it was: '*I will kick your saggy old ass.*' And I would laugh and then take another step, and another, and another. Because I did not want to die, and I did not want my old ass to be saggy anymore."

"But really, it was your honesty with me," she said. "When you said to do it or go away and die, I just knew it was true; it was one or the other. And my saggy old ass: That was like saying the leaves were falling off my tree, one by one, and I was losing my body, my life. And I knew you were right, just knew it deep down. You were right, so I took another step, and another. But the other amazing thing was that it took me nearly six months to look at myself in the mirror, and the day I was able to look myself in the eyes and, as you said, feel my love for me, well from that day on I have been pain free. Truly, not one bit of pain from that day. But I still smile at myself each morning so that is does not come back," she said, laughing.

Well to cut a long story short, June lived for another 12 years, fit, sprightly, trim (no saggy ass), no arthritis, no pain and no meds. She worked her garden, painted her house, travelled to Australia three times a year to see the grandkids, cooked, cleaned, looked after her beloved home, and died in her sleep after, as her daughter told me, the best, the most fun, the happiest 12 years of her life. And the day before she died, well into her 90s, she had done her three-mile walk, still without sticks and still laughing with joy. And her daughter told me that when she went to her mother's house and found she had passed, she could not stop looking at her. She said she looked so beautiful, her skin was smooth, and she looked just so happy.

You know, many times in my life when I hit brick walls and feel I can't do this or that anymore, or something seems way too hard to get through, my mind goes back to my friend, June. She did it beyond all odds. She just kept at it; she knew what was required and just did it. She could do it because she understood *how* it had happened in the first place. I had explained to her *what* took place in her body and *how* it got so toxic and painful. That was the knowledge that gave her the belief that she could reverse it and get her body and life back.

I share this story with you to show you that it is never too late, all is never lost, but most importantly, to encourage you to take ownership, to take responsibility for *you*. You see, there is really no disease. What we call disease is really an electrical malfunction of some group of cells. As the energy drops in the cells, for many reasons, the cells can't do what they are meant to do, and some function of the physical body starts to go haywire. What we call disease is the name given to that malfunction, or the physical manifestation of the electrical system overload or underload with-in those cells. And one of the biggest causes (other than chemical toxicity) of that energy blockage is emotional: our stress; our feeling unloved; our unhappiness with ourselves, our job, our partner, our relationship, or whatever. Just like we saw with June, when she got to the stage that she could look and really *see* and love herself, her pent-up emotions dissolved, her energy system charged up, her cells started to work again, her body recovered, and all her pain went away. Clean up the emotional energy, and the entire electrical system hums.

This being happy, not buying into others' emotional stuff, following and living your own truth, finding *you*, is the biggest factor to being healthy and beautiful. When you are happy, you glow; your skin reflects that inner joy and contentment. Your body's energy system charges up and every cell works better. Even your hormones are better-balanced. And God knows what we can be like when our hormones are out of balance. I have always said to all my women clients: "A healthy cell is a beautiful cell." Thus a healthy, fully-charged skin cell looks and feels beautiful.

So being healthy and looking and feeling beautiful is all about *you*, how you feel about you, and how you live this life in your body. But the responsibility is all yours. If you are not blissfully happy, change whatever is required to make you happy. An unhappy person will never have beautiful skin, never look fully alive, never walk around with that inner glow, and most of the time *will* be a right royal pain in the posterior to all those around them. Being unhappy will always put stress on your energy systems and thus lead to disease. I have found that cancer always has an emotional hook -- an emotional charge -- to it. As far as we know, we have only got this one experience in this one body, so you better not waste it being unhappy, or else, as I say: Go away and die! (oops, sorry Narah). Because being unhappy is just a waste of a life, your life. So change it.

June accepted the fact that 80 years of doing the wrong things to herself, 80 years of not knowing what was the right food, and 50 years of not really being happy in herself, nearly killed her in a miserable and painful way. But she owned it, took responsibility for her body, put the hard yards in, and got her body back, got her happiness back, got her life back, and looked and felt alive and beautiful. She just glowed with happiness and beauty. She found in herself the joy of being alive. She found herself, and everything changed.

June lived to show us all the reality and truth of *'ageless beauty'*.

4. HOW TO SLOW AGING

Most of us just see our body as nothing more than a thing that has to be fed, watered, and cleaned. We never -- well hardly ever -- give it another thought. But what is it, really? Yea, we somewhat know it is built of flesh, blood, and bone, and inside, it has all sorts of strange mechanisms: a pump, plumbing, filters, bellows, and lots of other stuff most of us never get to see or understand. And we know that it is all made up of cells. And that is about as far as most of our knowledge goes.

But what is a cell? Heck, what really is this *'thing'* called our body? Okay, let's go and find out, shall we?

We will start by going back, way back, right back to the core of our being. I could say we have to go back to the Sun, but even that would not be going back far enough. Even if I took you back to cosmic dust, that still would not be far enough. So where do we go from there? ENERGY.

Defining energy is a bit hard because it is something that we cannot see, feel, or touch. Well, that's not quite true either; we are seeing it, we are feeling it, and we are touching it. It's just that most people are not aware of it; their consciousness is just not developed -- or evolved -- enough to perceive it. As I explained earlier, some of us *can* see and *are* aware of much more than others, but that's another story.

What we call energy is actually hundreds of trillions of trillions of minute particles, fields of what we call current: impulses of light, electrons, and protons travelling at great speeds through time and space. The most costly science project ever undertaken, was put in place under the Swiss, French and German borders in a big round underground tunnel, in an effort to find the smallest part of energy. That science project is called CERN -- The European Organization for Nuclear Research -- and they crash the smallest particles of matter together in order to break them open to see what is inside. To date, the only thing they have found is even smaller bits, even more energy. Of course, this is really hard to do when you can't see what you are working with, because our eyes and our consciousness cannot even be aware of it. Yap, we still have a long way to go with this stuff called quantum science.

However, when these bits of 'light' or energy, slow down enough, they sort of condense, really just get slow enough for our consciousness to perceive, and we call that matter. I will say it another way: Take a piece of ice, some water and some air – nice, clean, fresh mountain air that contains 30% humidity. The ice, the water, and the humidity are all made of the same stuff: H_2O (that is two molecules of the gas we call Hydrogen and one molecule of Oxygen).

But ice, water, and humidity are very different things to us. If you were to jump into a block of ice from 50 meters, you would stand a good chance of killing yourself. A very sudden stop is in store for you. But if you jumped into a deep pool of water from the same height, it would be "Yee ha!" good fun with a big splash. But the humidity, hell, we don't even know it's there; we do not have any perception of it. But all three are made of exactly the same stuff. So what's the difference, and why is the same stuff -- the same three molecules -- seen, felt, and perceived by us differently?

It's because the vibrational rates, the *energy*, or the *frequencies* -- the speed of the protons and electrons moving inside the atoms -- are different. Take the ice: That stuff that we can see, feel and touch; it's real. Now, just for argument's sake, we will say that the bits in the atoms are moving at 100 miles per hour, round and around. At that speed it is solid (Well, to us at any rate). Now speed up the protons and electrons, and the ice becomes water; now the bits are running at 200 miles per hour. It's the same stuff, but by just changing the vibrational rate, the *frequency*, the speed of the bits, it is now very different and behaves differently. Water runs down the drain, but ice will not move. And how did we speed up the atomic bits? We gave them more *energy*: We heated them up, and heat *is* thermal energy. In a way, we just supplied more current and the bits got excited and ran around faster. A bit like when we give kids some energy in the form of sugar. Not too different, really. The same process is taking place in a way. Now let's speed up the protons and electrons even more, give them more current, more energy. Now they are going at 300 miles per hour. OMG! Now the stuff is gone; we cannot see it, can't feel it, and don't even know it is there! There is no ice; there is no water. Nothing! NOOO, it is still there, it's just that at that *frequency*, we cannot perceive it. Humidity is beyond our perceptional ability.

Look at this another way: The humidity, with its bits going at 300 miles per hour (using this just to get our head around it), is at a frequency that we cannot see. The old world called that the spirit world, or the *occult* which means "the unseen." And they were right; we now know things can be present and real even though we cannot see or know that they are there. Humidity is the perfect example. Now, let's slow down the *frequency*, take some energy out of the humidity -- cool it if you like. The bits in the atoms slow down, get closer together. As I said above, energy condenses as the protons and electrons get slowed down, and hey presto, we can now see, feel, and touch the stuff. We call it water. Take more energy out of it, slow down the atomic bits even more, slow down the vibrational rate, change the *frequency* and now it gets real dense: It's ice. Solid as a rock.

We have just performed a miracle. We have taken something that is tangible, something we can see, feel, and touch, and made it go into the spirit world outside of our ability to perceive, and then we brought it back to what we call our real world. And we did all that by just exciting, increasing the *frequency*, upping the energy and then taking the energy out again in a group of water (H$_2$0) molecules. Those molecules went from ice to water to something we cannot see and back to solid ice.

So now, listen up. Because this is where all this quantum physics stuff pertains to your body, your health, and your beauty. Every time we change the way nature works, take something out or put something into a mixture or product, or manipulate anything in any way, we change the atomic speed of the molecules. We change the *frequency*, the vibration rate -- the amount of *energy* -- that atom or group of molecules has, or is running at. Then we change its *action, reaction,* and *interface* with the rest of the universe. Drink that in: Your very life could depend on it.

Now you see, since our bodies are made of the same stuff as the rest of the universe, just a group of electrical fields called atoms grouped together to form molecules which make up our cells, it is fairly easy to see that if we introduce any form of energy into our cells, our cells MUST respond. Now, everything we hear, touch, smell, eat, apply to our skin, our emotions, feelings, moods, movement, in fact everything we do either brings us in energy or takes energy from us. And if we put enough stress on our cells -- lower the energy on enough cells or upset, distort, or block the energy -- disease must take place.

To tie all that in I want to explain just how energy flows through our cells and body. You have all seen that small thing-a-ma-jig (actually it's called a Newton's Cradle) that has about six steel balls hanging from it, all close together. You know that if you pull the end ball back away from the others and let it go, that ball swings down and hits the others. The balls in the middle do not move, but the ball on the other end swings out nearly as far as you pulled the first end one out.

The energy that was generated by the momentum of the ball as it swung down was transferred through the middle balls, and as the other end ball had no other ball to transfer its energy to, it was able to use that energy and swing out. Now, if you did the same thing, but this time held one of the middle balls between your fingers, then as you pulled out and let the end ball go, nothing, or very little would happen to the ball at the *other* end. You see, your fingers created an energy block, so no or very little, energy got transferred to the other end ball, so it could not do its thing and swing out. THIS IS THE SAME AS DISEASE. This is what happens to your cells before disease can be known or felt. There is an electrical malfunction, an *energy* block, a short circuit, an energy 'disruption', or an energy overload in a group of cells that stops the energy from flowing correctly to and through the cells. And if that low energy stays for long enough, or the energy in the cells gets low enough, then the cells physically malfunction and we have a disease.

This energy block can have many causes: emotions,

physical impacts, chemicals, antibiotics, preservatives, non-life-giving foods we eat, environmental toxins, stress, unhappiness. Just about everything we do, feel, eat, breath, or apply to our skin, can have and or cause electrical or *energy* issues in any cell in our body.

But that's not all. Our body is not an isolated object. It is not one stand-alone life form. Far from it. Our body is a farm and a garden. Critters live in you and on you; billions upon billions upon billions of living, breathing, breeding critters are crawling, munching, pooping, and living their lives all over every part of you, inside and outside. And they are made up of cells as well; they are energy as well, so we had better not upset their energy. You are awash with microbes, enzymes, and countless trillions of bacterial life forms. There is so much breeding going on inside of you it is mind boggling. Sometimes I think, "Wouldn't it be fun if we could be aware of all the sex taking place inside of us with those countless billions of critters? Darn, we would be in a state of orgasmic bliss 24/7!"

Sorry, the farm boy in me again. Just my twisted sense of humor.

But really, it's quite amazing when you think about it. We really *are* a walking farm and a garden. My good friend, Peter Baumann PhD., who is a retired head of research for one of the major pharmaceutical companies in Switzerland, told me that there are most likely more creatures living in and on us than there are cells in our body. Wow. Our digestive system alone contains by far the biggest farm -- huge herds of millions of micro bacteria and other critters. So you see, we do not live on the food we eat; we actually live on the poop of the tiny little critters inside us who eat that food.

"Denie, you can't say that, that's disgusting!"

Why not? It's the truth. It's how we get the good bits out of the food. You need to know this stuff, so you can think about the food you eat. Food has to feed the microbes before we get it. Why would I go into a big long scientific diatribe to explain the digestive process and how we get nourished using all the big long scientific words? Just to feed my ego or to justify the tens of thousands of dollars I spent on a higher education? Well, I don't have a higher education, so I don't have to pander to my ego. But I do know *how* this body works, and if I can pass that on to you so that you understand it, then you will know *how* your body works as well. Then you will know *how* to keep it healthy and beautiful. And if by saying just one word -- poop -- you get it, you understand perfectly what I mean and the process, then that's great. Way easier and quicker for us all, since it takes me hours to two-finger type all this stuff for you at any rate.

Sorry about that, just had to have a wee chat with myself. Let's proceed.

So, the micro bacteria and other critters eat the food, pass it through their little stomachs, and in the process break open the cell wall of the food and expose the protein molecule inside the cells of the food. That's the bit that goes through our stomach and intestinal wall into our blood. So without the farm of critters eating the food first and passing it through their digestive system and out you-know-where, we would starve. Digestion is the Latin word for *rotting*, and rotting is the process of bacterial breakdown. It's the same process that happens in a septic tank or in your city sewer plant. Now that's disgusting: to think we walk around with a septic tank inside of us. But it is the same process.

Another detail that none of the so-called health or diet books discuss is our flatulence (farts). But it is important to talk about, as it is a good way to know how your digestive system is working, a way to monitor if the critters inside are healthy and doing what they are meant to be doing: eating and pooping out the digested food we swallowed.

You see, everything that grows contains vitamins, minerals, proteins, fatty acids, amino acids, carbon, oxygen, nitrogen, and a whole host of other things that are required for life. When all this gets digested, or bacterially broken down, many gases are released including hydrogen, carbon dioxide, oxygen, nitrogen, and methane. Methane gas is 21 times more potent in the Earth warming equation than is CO_2, but due to its rather low concentration, it only adds about 7% to the total equation. (Okay, just thought you should know that your (or the animals') farts don't cause Earth warming).

Since all mammals, including us, have this big digestive process going on inside, we produce gas. Well, it's not us really; it's all those billions and billions of feeding critters in our gut. So if good digestion produces gas, then we can gauge how our gut is working by the gas production. As we all know, when we eat really easy-to-digest foods like grapes, cherries, and other fruits, we feel we produce more gas. That's not so much the case; it's just that our farm workers inside were able to get the job done faster, and the gas was produced in a shorter time frame, and thus had to be passed in bigger bubbles more often.

So in a way, we can tell if our digestive system is working, tell if the critters are doing their job, or more to the point, if we are giving them the right food with the most life force, by our farts. The easier the food breaks down for the critters, the more life force we get from it. So when you have a good, odorless fart, rub your belly and thank the critters for doing a good job in keeping you healthy, energetic, and nourished. Now, if your farts carry a bad odor (yap, we have all been there), that is telling us, "Wrong food, wrong combination." For good digestion, and to make life way easier for the farm workers inside -- and remember if it wasn't for them you would die -- it is always better *not* to combine protein and carbohydrates in the same meal. If you keep to protein and veggies without the carbs, your farts will never have an odor, and the farm will work way better, and you will have way more energy, and your skin will also look much more beautiful. Carbs are one of the hardest for the farm to deal with and they do *not* give you energy. This carb-energy craze is the biggest bull ever sold. From a biological and digestive-science standpoint, it doesn't work. All carbs do is screw up your hormones, fatten you up, dull your skin tone, irritate your bowels, make smelly farts, and lower your energy. And that's a fact. We haven't had bread, cakes, cereal, cookies or any crude carbs in our house for over 20 years. And at 67 years of age, I will take on any carb-eating, 30-something and whip his you-know-what every time.

Another story: When I was a very little lad, my dad still had horses to do some of the farm work. Each morning he used to go out to the horse paddock and walk the three horses around for a bit. Well, we kids soon learned why he did that. The horse that farted the most was the one he harnessed up for the day's work. True story. (Stop laughing; it really is true!)

And here is why: The horse that was feeling good, had no pain, and was fit and healthy would have eaten a belly full of grass the day before (no animal eats if it is not feeling well); therefore, it had a lot of digestion going on, and there was a lot of gas produced. And you all know only too well that when you first move in the morning, your body evacuates the gas. You fart. So the horse that farted the most was the one that would have had the most energy to work hard that day -- that was the one that Dad harnessed up. Simple, eh?

I remember a little saying I got from my Uncle Lew who took over Grandad's farm in South Taranaki. He used to say it when one of us kids let one go at the breakfast table or whatever: "A farting horse will never tire, a farting man is the one to hire." Okay, okay, but in so many ways, so true. It really does explain or give an insight to the fact that the old timers new a thing or two about nature. Heck, they had to, their livelihoods depended on knowing how nature worked.

Oh, and another saying that Uncle Lew used to crack us cousins up with was when one of us kids let go (you know what) and Aunty would give us 'that look', but Uncle would laugh and say to us kids: "When you hold your farts in, they slide up your back bone and into your brain and give you shitty thoughts." We young'uns just loved old Uncle Lew, especially us boys. So there you go; now you know the deep and meaningful philosophy on life of my old Uncle Lew. Oh dear, you can take the boy out of the farm, but you can never take the farm out of the boy. ☺

Right you lot, get yourselves together again. Let's move on, shall we? So to slow this aging process down, you need to understand how this body works, and the biggest and most important part of the entire system is your stomach, your digestion. Because that is the only place you get fed from, nourished from, and your life force from. You all know how you feel when your gut goes haywire: Not good. Every part of your body goes into decline when your gut can't give you what you need. Your skin tone -- the look of your skin -- is almost directly indexed to how your gut is working.

The first thing we old farmers look at in our animals each day is their skin tone -- or rather the look and condition of their coat (their hair). The look of their coat will always give us the best and earliest warning if something is amiss with our animals. And it is the same with us people. Therefore, if you are not happy with your skin, look at what you are putting into and onto your body. Because if you put anything into or onto your body (and chemical skin creams are by far the worst), that does not give or enhance life, you will be putting a stress on the energy fields of the cells and causing the cell energy to drop. Your life force will go down, and you will look and feel like, well, you know the word.

One last short story. I have to share this with you, because this chapter is about slowing down the aging process. My oldest cow, back when I was farming 500 milking cows in New Zealand, was old 91 (the number of her ear tag was her name as well). She was 105 years old by human equivalent. Living outside and eating natural grass all her life, she was still able to get pregnant, calve unassisted, and milk for 10 months. And she had not missed a season, ever (91, as with all animals had the same biological process as we do). So I think I know a thing or two about how to slow down this aging process. I know a thing or two, because I have seen a thing or two; and I have seen a thing or two, because I have done a thing or two, including 30 years helping thousands of clients get their health, their beauty, and their lives back. So let's move on, shall we, and find out *how*.

.

5. ANTI-AGING FOOD

Surprisingly, when I look at people, I see very few who look really healthy and full of life. Yet there must be more books, more information, more supplements, more fads, more advice, and more so-called nutritional experts than ever before in human history. So why aren't we all just bursting with health, vigor, and vitality? Why are we not satisfied with the way we look? Why do we still feel the need to mask our dull-looking skin with makeup every day before we leave the house?

Maybe, just maybe, most of the information out there is 90 percent BS. Maybe the nutritional advice is not what it should be. But how can we measure, really, what is happening to our vitally, to our life force? Look, in agricultural science, we know that one of the best parameters to gauge the life force or vitality in our animals is the sperm count of the young bulls. Since the 70s, when we figured this out, we have monitored the young bulls coming into New Zealand's dairy breeding program, so that we know the ups or downs of their sperm count. We know that this should not drop more than three percent from the base line; otherwise, we have a problem with the life force and health of the national herd. Since that time, New Zealand has been able to keep the sperm count in this three percent range. In other words, we have been able to keep our animals with the same or better healthiness and life force for over fifty years with no drop off in overall vitality, health, or ability to breed.

Now let's look at how we, as humans, stack up. About 25 years or so ago, when I first came to America, I inspired a program as a result of a public talk I gave in Wenatchee, Washington. A group of doctors instigated a program to test the sperm count of the local high school boys -- 15 to 17-year-olds. Now to get a good, accurate count, the semen needs to be as fresh as possible. As one of the doctors said to me afterwards: "The table of plastic beakers we had ready for the lads to deposit their samples in was bare in about five seconds."

The mind boggles to think what was going through the heads of those lads at the time: "Really, I can do this in the name of science, really, where is that beaker?"

Suffice to say, there was no shortage of very willing volunteers. I still chuckle at the thought of a bunch of high school lads doing their 'thing' to further humanity's scientific knowledge. Way to go lads.

However, those boys' testosterone-driven feelings of manhood soon took a tumble. The results that came back showed that, overall, the sperm count was nearly 70% below the 1948 level, and in fact 20% of the samples were so low that, medically, they would be classified as infertile.

Heck, I had stirred up a real hornet's nest in the community, because when the results were published there were public meetings called, the school board was held over the coals for not having enough protein and real nutrition in the school lunch program, there was a small group of mothers who held a protest outside the local supermarket to demand more real, alive and organic food, all sorts of things. I had done my job; time to leave town, so I did.

Since that time the American Medical Association (AMA) has also published findings that back up the Washington results. Knowledge is now in the public domain that the sperm count of the average, young, white, American male is 70% below the 1940's level. Just drink that in people. More than *half* the life force, health, and vitality, to say nothing of the ability to breed, has disappeared from the general public. And if you don't believe me, CNN recently reported the following: "The US fertility rate fell to the lowest point since record keeping started more than a century ago, according to statistics released by the Centers for Disease Control and Prevention."

Some months later, I was invited to give a talk on natural health and how the body works electrically to a large gathering of somewhat enlightened, rather young doctors on the east coast -- about 200 or so of them. Of course, I used the sperm count example as part of my presentation. At the end of my talk I finished with these words:

"You have all listened to me, a mere farm boy from New Zealand, talk about health and vitality and how this body works from a different angle. However, you all have a higher level of education in the science of health. And your core mission - the reason you are, or intended to become, doctors is to give your advice to, and to help maintain or improve the health and lives, of the people. If you in this room are so good at what you do, and your science is so good, and you know your stuff, why is it then that none of you are half the men your grandfathers were?"

Oh my God, you could have heard a pin drop. Dead silence for some time. Then an older doctor from near the back of the room stood up and clapped.

He then said: "You are right, Farm Boy. We need to hear and take in your message and we, as a medical profession, need to take a hard long look at ourselves."

Well with that the whole room, to a person, stood up and I got a standing ovation. I sometimes think back to that day and smile. Gee, my science, my logic, and my message got through to them, all of them. And I was probably the only one in that room without a PhD.

So what is it that gives us this life? Yap, oxygen is important. Deny our body of oxygen for more than three or four minutes and most of us are out of here. Sunlight, yap: If that huge thermonuclear thing wasn't happening in our neighborhood none of us would be here either. But by far the most life-giving thing we do is eat. FOOD people: glorious food. And a tad (that's a 'small bit' for you non-Kiwis) of chocolate. Well maybe not so small; it is chocolate after all.

Food. Digestion. We all know these words and now I hope you got your head around this digestion process as well. Remember: We do not get nourishment directly from food. That's right: It's bacterial breakdown by the farm critters inside us. If we only get our life force from the food that the critters digest for us first, then we had better make darn sure we put into our stomachs, that which the critters can easily eat.

Raw fresh fruit is way up there on the scale of good foods, but here is the best way to know what is the most available food we can eat. Since digestion is a rotting process, put the food you are going to eat on your kitchen counter and leave it at room temperature for five to seven days. The food that starts to rot in that time will be the most available to you for your life force, give you the most energy, and thus beauty.

"How is that?" you ask.

The air all around us is also loaded with molds, yeast, and countless bacteria. So if you leave food out, the critters in the air, as well as the ones living in the food, start to have a feast.

"Oooh," you say. "Bacteria in the food?"

Yes, as I said earlier, all living beings are walking farms and gardens of some sort; everything is alive, teaming with sub-microscopic life. It's called nature. It's simple: What the critters outside your body can break down in five to seven days at room temperature, the farm critters inside your stomach can do in three hours (that's all the time they have, due to our short digestive tract). Why? Because there is acid in our stomach which helps dissolve the wax wall of the food cells, and it is very moist and at the perfect temperature for the billions of critters to multiply, so there are enough to properly do the job. Also, you might have *lightly* cooked it, to help break open the cell walls, and hopefully chewed it up lots (broken open some more cells) and covered it with saliva, all helping the process.

So what rots on the counter in a week? Raw meat, raw eggs out of their shell, fish, raw milk, ripe fruit, berries, unprocessed cheese, etc. All the protein foods that were once alive and breathing. Really, all the raw, or slightly cooked, unprocessed protein from nature as well as ripe fruits and berries.

Think about it: Not much else goes rotten in a week. Does grain (seeds)? Never. In fact there is not a single critter that will eat grain for food. Look, leave some breakfast cereal out on the counter. Hell, in 10 years it will still be there. No critter in the world will eat it and pass it through its digestive tract. If the critters will not eat it, how the hell do you think it can be food for you? In fact, no seeds are eaten by anything for food on this earth, except us non-thinking (totally misinformed) humans. Also, does much vegetation go rotten in a week on the counter? NO! It might dry out, but it is untouched by the critters. A carrot will not decay in weeks, if ever. Okay, I have explained this thing about grain in my two earlier books, *Electrical Nutrition* and also in *A Little Book of Wisdom*, so I will not do it again. But just to hit it home to you I will say again the farmer's mantra: "Grain for gain, protein for production."

Think on that. If you want to get fat, toxic, have low energy, screw up your hormones, and give yourself bad skin, pimples, emotional swings, thyroid problems, diabetes, bowel disease, and destroy every joint in your body (arthritis), it's easy: Just eat a lot of grain-based so-called food. Anything made from a seed or ground up seeds (also known as flour), is *not* food. Bread, pasta, cereal, burger buns, cookies, you know; the crap you all eat every day? IT IS NOT FOOD.

Neither is Soy. Soy milk is *not* food (and I have never seen a soy cow, have you?); it is Soy Protein Isolate, and that is a toxic non-food. It has not even received "GRAS" status (generally recognized as safe) by the Food and Drug Administration (FDA). In fact, New Zealand's health department issues public health warnings on soy products on national TV. Soy products will screw your hormones and can severely affect young women's ability to get pregnant. Furthermore, it is a neuro-toxin that can blast your emotions all over the universe. Feeding soy milk to young girls can even stop their reproductive organs from developing. In my book, *Electrical Nutrition*, I published the full "Soy Science

Report." Read it, and then tell me that soy is a food. Also, soy is the *most* genetically modified (GMO) plant ever to be grown. There is not a non-GMO modified soy plant grown; they do not exist anymore. Soy milk and other Soy Protein Isolate products do not contain any semblance to nature's life-giving energy or vibrational symphony. None. It is a man-made abomination sold to the health food wannabes *in order to dispose of the toxic remains* after the good bit of the soy plant has been extracted to make Soya sauce.

Another myth: whey is a digestible food. NOT. If whey protein was digestible, it would have been digested by the starter bacteria and enzymes in the cheese making process. Whey is used in most protein drinks and sometimes only labeled as milk protein. In my book, *A little Book of Wisdom*, I give the full science of whey. But trust me: it is *not* a digestible food protein.

Now, back to the grain story. Your body, your farm, *cannot* process grain into a usable form of energy. It cannot get, or extract, the protein bit, which is the only bit your body wants and needs to sustain your life or your health in the short time it is in your system. That's why God gave a cow four stomachs, a 72-hour digestive system, and the ability to grind her food *twice*, at five thousand pounds-per-square-inch pressure. And she only gets 20% of the available nutrition out of young grass in that process -- what we would call veggies for us. She gets *slow* and *fat* (just like us) when we give her grain. Her production (and her production is the gauge for her health and life-force) goes *down* when we give her too much grain, *not up*. This is not a debate: IT IS BIOLOGY, pure and simple.

God (nature) made a seed to germinate in order to grow the next generation of thin-walled cells of what are correctly called *herbs,* which literally means *edible vegetation*. For that to happen, the seed was designed to *never* be broken down by being eaten by the micro critters in the air, in the ground, or in the stomach of anything. The seed had to stay intact on the ground, pass through the stomach of birds and not be digested, so as to be able to germinate and grow the young grasses and spread the trees, etc., in the next growing season. If seeds could be broken down by rotting or digestion, then there would be no greenery on Earth. God (nature) *did not* make a seed for food. And *anybody* who tries to tell you that grain (seeds) or grain-based food is *food*, DOES NOT EVEN KNOW OR UNDERSTAND A DARN THING ABOUT BASIC BIOLOGY, and, furthermore, shows a complete and total lack of knowledge and understanding of what digestion is, or *how* it works. End of story.

Yes, I hear some of you yelling from the tree tops: "But the old cultures ate grain!"

Yes, that's right. But *never* in the way we eat it today. In times of old, in times of famine, when there was little other protein available, the seeds were collected, crushed, and the outer layers were allowed to blow away in the wind (Heck they even knew that the outer fibers were no good and let them blow away. Today we get told that 'whole' grain is good. NOT. The outer fibers are devastating to our bowel health), then the bit inside the seed, the bit that held the *'germ'* or the bit of the seed that contained the protein, was ground up and then mixed with raw milk into a paste. The milk was usually given by the lactating mums of the tribe or milked from their sheep or goats. The live enzymes and good bacteria in the milk were the starter for the digestion process. In this case, the mixed, ground-up seeds and milk paste were put in the hot sun and allowed to ferment (digest or be eaten and pass through the stomach of the millions of critters) for up to 14 days. Yes, 14 days. This, then, extracted (made available) the protein from the seed fibers and the *'germ'* of the seed. That ferment was then mixed with some vegetation, herbs, spices, etc., and fed to the hungry kids. So they only ate pre-digested – fermented -- seeds which now contained some available protein. Never in human history was grain eaten as we do today -- as crude or refined carbohydrate. The way we eat grain today is not food and can (will) cause all the issues and diseases outlined above.

We have been told a lie about grain-based food, because it does not spoil (nothing will eat it), so it lasts a long time in the shops. It doesn't get contaminated in the processing and packing plants; it's easy and cheap to store, so it is easy to make a *profit* from it. *And* every scientist knows full well it will cause many of the most profitable diseases we suffer from today. *Get it?* Need I say any more? Think about it: There is *no* expiration date on a packet of breakfast cereal. It will never spoil, so it's okay to sell it 10 years after it was harvested. If nothing will eat it, then doesn't that tell you it is DEAD, that no life can be extracted from it (and you feed that toxic, life-destroying non-food 'stuff' to your kids!)? Blimey, if the micro critters won't even eat it, one must ask, why do you? Since it's only the eating of food by the critters in your stomach that gives YOU life, NOTHING ELSE. Can I suggest that the critters have more brains and intelligence than we do? It would seem so, WAKE UP people.

And I repeat for all of you that have short attention spans from eating way too much grain based non-foods: We have a short digestive process, so we only get a small portion of the nutrition available from vegetation, and like *all* other animals, we get *nothing* out of the seed. Oh, except fat, toxic and screwed up with bad skin and most of the other biological diseases mentioned above. *We,* and other animals, were never intended, never designed, to eat grain or grain-based 'stuff' as food. God's rules - not mine. I did not design this thing called life, or digestion, I am just trying to show you, *how* it works.

Now, if anything is processed, cooked too much, contains preservatives, or is changed from the way nature made it, it will not have the correct -- or fully charged -- electrical fields around the molecules; therefore, the transfer to you as life-giving will be compromised. Also, the energy field from any food drops off each day from the day it was harvested. For instance, an organically grown carrot will lose 50% of its life force in 14 days from harvest. Remember, it's all about energy. We do not actually get life from the food we eat; we get our life from the *energy* of the food -- that subtle field of energy, those protons and electrons running around inside of the atoms. Life is all about the transfer of energy. Remember, the thingy (Newton's Cradle) with the swinging balls? Right, anything we do to live food, *anything*, is like putting our fingers on one of the middle balls. It stops or slows the *energy* transfer.

Also, there is very little vegetation on Earth that is able to be eaten by our farm critters in the three hours that they have to process our food as it passes through our system. Everything alive is built from protein and fats. Our bodies are all protein and fats, and to be nourished we need available protein and the good fats. Yes, vegetation has protein, but our farm critters cannot get to it quickly enough to digest and open its cells, so it cannot nourish us much. It's not a debate about vegetarianism; it's just simple biology and an eating process by the farm workers in our gut.

Therefore, the most effective anti-aging foods are those that contain readily-available protein and the good fats, which is all animal protein and most fruits and berries with easily-broken-down, soft cell structures, eaten as close to harvest time as possible. However, deep freezing can maintain a near-to-raw life force level, if flash frozen within hours of harvest.

One of the most interesting observations is the difference between the people in Europe and those in the USA. In the USA, close to 60% are fat, toxic, and slow. Also, in the USA, over 60% of the population is on medication of some sort. In Europe, about 20% are on meds, and, generally speaking, people walk so much faster, are leaner and more vibrant, with only 10% obesity. Their skin is glowing, looks vibrant and they use far less make-up. The life force difference is profound. But really, the two groups eat much the same foods; however, in Europe, the time from harvest to plate is about two weeks, and in the village areas of Spain, rural France, Eastern Europe and Switzerland it can get down to four days. In America, it is up to six weeks. I will never understand the stupidity of Florida oranges in California supermarkets, and California oranges in Florida supermarkets.

Remember what I said about the drop in *energy* of the food after harvest. So Americans have to eat two or more times the food to try to be nourished as do their European cousins. All that dead, low-energy food that the Americans eat that can't be utilized for energy, because it has none, gets stored as congealed pus in their bodies. You call it *cellulite*. Also, because digestion uses the most energy of any process in the body, Americans have less energy to use for living, because a lot more is being used to try to process all that extra low-energy food, thus: slow, fat, toxic, people. However, it's interesting to note that in California, the state that grows about a third of the food in America, the people get some of their food with a shorter harvest-to-plate time, and California has one of the lowest ratios of fat-toxic people in the nation.

As a side note, all food in Europe has to be labeled with the *harvest* date, not just the *expiration* date, on the labels. Even eggs have the harvest date stamped on every one, so the consumer knows how old it is. And to them, fresh is best. Also in Europe, there is a huge move toward locally-grown food. Restaurants and hotels advertise and promote their 'locally grown' kitchens. In America, food is labeled with an expiration date. That is, how long it will last with all the preservatives in it. And that could be months. Our life force, that energy we have for life, comes not only from food's calorific value, but also, and mainly, from the electrical charge of the food -- the energy it has. This thing we call life is all based on *energy*.

Thus anti-aging food is, as much as possible, raw or prepared with minimal cooking, food that is easily broken down by the micro-bacteria in your gut -- food that rots quickly if you like: Animal protein, the good fats (from animals), most fruits and berries, avocados etc., with some veggies to help the elimination process. NO grain and minimal other carbs. Simple. And eat whole milk yogurt, but never reduced fat or non-fat milk or yogurt. God (nature) put the perfect Omega 3 - Omega 6 ratio of good fats in all mammal's milk. To think that low-fat or non-fat natural foods are good, is saying God (nature) got it wrong. Not. Only we (non-thinking humans) got it wrong.

A short story about the power of food -- the right food -- with the most energy in it: Some years ago a client was brought to my clinic in Switzerland. She had to be helped up the short flight of stairs by two others. She was the most emaciated, skinny, suicidal, and sick human I have seen, and I have seen a lot. It wasn't a question of whether she had a month or two to live; she was on her way out in days, if not hours. Nothing was working in her body, and she was in total emotional shock. She could not even put words together to make a sentence. Truly one of the sickest people, if not the sickest, I have ever seen still able to take a breath. The doctors had told her about a year before that she had auto-immune disease (in my experience that is the name given when they have no idea what is going wrong), and that she would not live long at all -- that there was nothing they could do.

I will skip all the unnecessary details, but I worked for three days in a row on her energy system to get some semblance of life into the poor creature. We got her to the point she could at least stand -- just barely -- without support, and a very slight bit of color came back to her skin. I mean, you have never seen a more-deathly-white person still breathing. When my time in that clinic was up and I had to leave for the U.S. again, I had to figure out what I could recommend for her to eat. The problem was that her body rejected all food; she just threw everything back up. As I said, her body had shut down; she was dying -- and quickly.

As I had gotten some charge back into her system with my energy work and most of the circuits somewhat working, and had put some space between the woman and her grave, I had to think what nutrition her body could absorb.

This is what I did. I organized with her caregiver to go to

the local village butcher and get him to cut the leg bones of the young, grass-fed Alp cows and scrape out the bone marrow. I gave instructions that she was to eat the raw bone marrow mixed with a small amount of raw cream (slightly heated to body temp) from the Alp farms, and she was to be fed a small amount of that each hour she was not sleeping. Or at least four or five times day. We started her out on one teaspoon-full each time, and slowly increased it as her energy came back. I also said that as she gained strength, she could eat some Alp wild berries or organic cherries and Alp cheese, but only as and if she felt like it. She got to the stage she was able to eat about a cupful of marrow with about half-a-cup of cream a day. And that was all she needed because of the electrical, or energy transfer, power in the marrow and the raw essential fatty acids in the cream, which has the most perfect omega 3 and 6 ratio for us humans. And none of it was more than a day or two from harvest. God did not get it wrong.

Cut to six months later when I returned to Switzerland. Up the stairs and in walked this still-very-skinny, but not the see-through-skinny woman of six months before. A smile on her face and *very* much alive. I was given the biggest, longest hug I have ever been given. I could hardly believe it, even though I was looking at her. She was so much more alive but still had a long way to go. But what a turn around. Now that she had enough energy, enough life force in her body, I could go in and get her electrical system all up and running and start to deal with her emotional baggage. The actual cause of her illness was total emotional sadness, a cell energy loading that was squeezing the very life out of her (another long story), but over the next two years we got her healthy and able to fully function, walk for hours in the mountains, and rejoin the work force.

She ate nothing other than the bone marrow and the raw cream for that six months, and over time we were able to reintroduce other good food into her system: colostrum; fresh Alp yogurt; cheese; butter; good, fresh, grass-fed meat; more berries; and a small amount of veggies. To this day NO grain-based, non-food has passed her lips. You see, the raw bone marrow had, within it, all the electrical fields needed for life -- all the energy transfer factors, all the minerals, all the protein, all the right fats, all the essential fatty acids -- everything, in the perfect ratios, and almost no digestion was needed because it was already digested. It was pure life -- pure energy -- because bone marrow is the body's energy bank, if you like. It was better than feeding her mother's milk. However, if raw colostrum had been available, she would have drunk that as well. So there you go: Almost all healing, coupled with the right energy rewiring and energy work, can be achieved with the right nourishment, the right food. I could not have turned that woman around if I did not know *how* this thing we call a body worked, and by knowing the *how* we were able to help this young lady (and many more thousands over the years), get her body back, her life back. As a side note, she is still very much alive today. So much for what medical folk know, or don't.

6. AGELESS BEAUTY

Time, for all of us, marches on from the day we are born. However, our body starts to feel and show the effects of time before any of us wants it to. Time, we can do nothing about, but the effect on how we look and feel with time is totally in our control. It is up to us. Period. So, if that's the case, and we are not happy with our lack of "ageless beauty," we had better get to it and do something about it.

So let's start with skin. Our glorious skin: It's the first bit any of us feels and sees each day. It's the first bit of us everybody else sees also. So what is it, really? And how do we keep it looking ageless and beautiful?

Our skin is the biggest organ of our body, and an organ can be loosely described as a life-support mechanism. Also, the skin is an absorbable membrane, similar to our stomach lining. Substances can go through it and come out of it. It is a living, breathing membrane and like the

59

rest of our body, our skin is host to a farm and a garden. That is, it is teeming with micro bacteria and all the other critters that are living in and on it to keep us healthy and alive. Remember, our body is not this stand-alone '*thing*', but rather it is a biological life form made up of countless trillions of different life forms, each with a job to do and all working in harmony to keep the whole healthy and alive. Change any of the parameters of any part of that complicated life process, and we are setting ourselves up for trouble.

Therefore, it is not rocket science to understand that if we put anything on our skin that has the capacity to kill, or in some way to interfere with the biological process taking place on or in our skin, we are setting ourselves up for disease, or at least some form of life shutdown. It has to happen.

Our skin cells, as with every cell in our body, in fact, every cell of every critter, those countless trillions of micro life forms that are living in and on us, respond to everything we do, eat, and apply. Think about that. *Everything* we do, eat, every emotion, and every skin cream, sun cream, or lotion we apply has to have an effect. The cells *either gain life* from what we do, or life is *taken away* by what we do or apply. *Every cell of us, every cell of the countless trillions of life forms living in and on us, either gains life or loses life as a direct result of our actions.* There is no grey bit in the middle somewhere where nothing happens. Truly, it is either giving life or taking life. Period. And our health, happiness, and beauty are governed by that, are *totally* indexed to that. Drink that in people. Drink that in. Now, think on this: Do your chemical skin creams, your sun blocks, your eye creams, etc., go rotten in a week? No way; they last for years, and nothing eats them. In other words: They cannot support life. So why in God's name would you put them on the living farm that is your skin? It will kill the farm that is you, and most of the chemicals will transfer through to your blood.

Now let's look at all this from an energy understanding, an electrical perspective. In my book, *Electrical Nutrition*, I stated that this thing we call a body is governed by, and supports, about a hundred million electrical impulses per second. My good friend, Peter Baumann, PhD (mentioned earlier), who is one of the top scientists in Europe, after reading my book, said to me that I was not quite accurate on that point. He said: "If you took your hundred million impulses per second to the power of 10, then you would be closer to the actual level." Think on that all you math and numbers folks: a hundred million to the power of ten. WOW. It's truly a mind-blowing number of electrical impulses, or bits of energy, flying around inside our bodies every second.

Knowing this, and as I have said many times, this life, the functioning of this body of ours, is an electrical -- or energy -- process, as is everything in the universe. Electrical impulses, are *how* every atom that comprises this thing we call our body, gets, understands, and knows *what* to do and *how* to function.

How is that possible? You ask. How does an electrical

impulse, a flow of energy, tell our cells *what* to do and *how* to work? First you need to grasp the fact that *all energy* contains all the necessary information to function correctly. It works just like the field of energy, the energy wave, the sound waves, or the transmission of a TV signal works -- how it brings the information to your TV. If you go outside and look up in the air, you do not see the Kardashians or CNN float on by. No, you see only sky. However, going through the air are impulses of electrical energy waves that are transmitted from the TV station. The sound and the visual pictures are made into electrical impulses and are transmitted out, and your TV aerial receives -- is calibrated to -- these vibrations of energy impulses. The circuits and processes in your TV turn on different frequencies of energy in the light or energy receptors in the TV screen, and then you can see the picture and hear the sound.

So everything, all information, can be made into an energy impulse. That is what happens with our eyes, our brain, our nerves, and it is how all information is transmitted to every atom in our body. So yes, all the information is sent around our body as a form of energy. Even our food transmits its information to our cells by an energy impulse. In reality, very little of the actual physical bit of what food *is* gets into our cells, and none of it gets into the atoms that the cells are made of. It is only the energy that gets transmitted and acted upon. By changing the frequency of the impulse, the cells can perform their different functions and, in fact, can become different cells. Change the vibrational fields, the energy, within a cell and the cell changes to a different action, becomes a different cell: A skin cell can become a heart cell, a blood cell can become a bone cell, etc. In fact, when we understand this, there is no need to use stem cells or any other expensive physical process to heal or in fact to grow new limbs or new organs. No need for organ transplants. Just by changing the *frequency* of the energy impulse we can get any cell to become a different cell in the body, to change its function.

How do I know this? I see it. It's how my outer fields of consciousness presents information to my brain -- how the universe presents itself to me; If you think that's strange, you should try living in this body, this mind, of mine. Sadly, the medical world, and big pharmaceutical companies, are too invested in their profits from drugs and surgeries, to allow -- yes allow -- any university or group of people to put money and time into understanding how the body works from an energy, or electrical, basis. And if they did, they would soon be shut down, none of their findings would be made public, no media would bring it to the general public's attention, and in the worst case, the people involved would simply disappear, or die an untimely death with some mysterious circumstance.

Now, back to the Kardashians on our TV screen: The TV needs to get *all* the energy impulse information. To hear a song on the radio, or whatever, it needs to get all the information; to have a pleasant tune we need to hear all the notes in the right places and in the right order and also with the right spaces between the notes. Otherwise, the tune would not sound harmonious. You see, our cells do not know what the individual notes on their own mean; they only get life from the *symphony* of energy. They need *all* the information with the right timing in order to act or react.

Now, as everything is and has an energy charge to it, that energy wholeness has to be available to the cells for the cell to know *what* to do and *how* to work. Therefore, if we give, put on, or do anything to our body that does not contain nature's vibrational field, nature's *symphony* of life in perfect harmony, what the body knows as life-giving or can recognize as containing the energy of life itself, then the cells cannot get the information that is needed for correct function. Without this natural symphony, or the energy wholeness, an energy distortion *will* take place, which can crash the energy fields in the cells and cause disease or even death. This is what the bye-bye drug, the one that the vet gave to our old horse, Sam, did. The drug did not put Sam to sleep, as he was dead before the drug got anywhere in his body. It was an electrical distortion -- a short circuit caused by the energy field of the chemicals that were the drug, the non-life-giving frequency, or the extremely distorted, foreign frequency, of the vibrational fields of the chemicals -- that totally crashed the horse's energy system. No energy, no life. Energy wise, the drug was like an electrical napalm bomb hitting the energy system of old Sam. That extremely unnatural energy frequency of the drug knocked out the life energy of Sam, and in that split second (energy is just the same as light, so it travels at the speed of light), he was dead.

"Quantum physics," you say.

Darn right this is quantum physics. This is how the universe works, and as we are a part of the universe, built on the same principles as the universe, made of the same stuff as the universe, we *are* the universe. Thus, we are energy.

This chapter is about ageless beauty, and to most of us, beauty is how our skin looks and feels. So let's look at that from an energy perspective. Our skin is not just this thin, leaky, leather-like encasement that holds all the other bits of our body from falling out all over the place. But rather, it is, as is the rest of our body, a living biological farm made up of billions of unseen critters. It is a large, interconnected group of cells -- cells made up of atoms, which are all vibrating fields of energy. Some of which are quite still, like our skin atoms, and some are rushing all over the place like the critters that are living *in* and *on* our skin. Also, now you know that this energy that is us, and our skin, responds to everything we experience, everything we do, everything we touch, everything we eat, and everything we put onto it. Because all energy responds and interacts with all other energy.

We have also learned, that this energy field that is us, and our skin, has evolved to know and recognize what the symphony of life is. In fact, when it is all working right and in complete harmony, it *is* the harmonic symphony of life. This symphony of perfect life is called *homeostasis*, not only of our cells but also of the critters living in and on us as well. We are not separate; our life is their life and vice versa.

Therefore, in order to have our skin looking and feeling as we want it to, we had better put on it only that which also contains the perfect symphony of life, or, in simple terms, that which evolved with us, what we call *natural*. Because anything unnatural cannot have the right energy fields of life -- the correct symphony. Also, as there are billions of critters living in and on our skin, we had better not put anything on our skin that damages or adversely affects their ability to function, live, and to do their jobs of keeping that part of us alive and healthy.

That said, humans have spawned an industry, to the tune of twenty billion dollars annually, whose only reason for existence is to feed our genetic urge to look and feel beautiful. Our genetic urge is not wrong; in fact, as stated earlier, it is an honorable cause, a necessary urge, and a powerful one at that. But the skin care industry responded to that powerful urge without any thought as to *what*, nor *how,* our bodies, our cells, our energy systems might respond to, or be damaged by, its products. We have slapped, slopped, and plastered creams and lotions on our living, highly populated skin with never a thought about the long-term effects.

Really, how could we know? We were never told that this body, and our skin, has this amazing life to it. We were never told that most products we put on our skin would kill the farm on our skin and end up in our blood. We were never told that this thing called a body is a finely-tuned vibrational field of energy that can easily be knocked out of harmony, out of homeostasis, by things that do not contain the fields of energy that evolved in our natural bubble of life.

Remember the ice, water, and humidity lesson? If we change the frequency of anything, we change its action, reaction, and interface with everything else. Therefore, if we manipulate the molecules of any substance, natural or not, we will change the energy fields of the resulting product, and with that it will be unlikely to have any life-giving vibrations, no harmonic symphony of life. It will be what we term *toxic* to life, or at best, non-life-giving. And as I said earlier: If something does not give life, it takes away life.

Our entire skin care industry, the one that we have trusted and empowered over the last 50 years has, by and large used a manipulation called chemistry to take apart known cancer-causing compounds, mainly crude oil molecules (where petrochemicals come from) and reassemble them to make different chemicals to sell as skin care products. Why? Because oil molecules are very slippery and when applied to our skin make it feel nice and soft. These chemicals still contain some of the energy fields that cause cancer and when reassembled have NO energy or vibrational match with life in any way. In fact, when applied to our skin, they not only kill the critters living in and on our skin, but they also have a similar, though slower, effect to the energy napalm bomb that happened to my horse, Sam.

Therefore, to get our skin to that beautiful, youthful, and ageless look and feel we all so desire, we must put compounds on our skin that are truly natural in all ways and that also contain the electrical -- or energy -- vibrations of life and feed and give life to the farm that is living on our skin. Natural oils, which many people use on their skin, can very often suffocate the critters, as they do not allow oxygen through. Also, many natural compounds, like bee's wax and lanolin, do not support life. Bee's wax is used to seal toilets to the drain so that no bacteria can get back into our houses, because bee's wax kills *all* microbes. That's why bees use it to build their houses: so nothing will eat the house. Bee's wax will not decay in a 1000 years, so it does not promote healthy skin. Understanding that, why would anyone want to use a bee's wax-based lip product? Our lips are teeming with life; the critters living on our lip tissue have a very important job to do. They are the first line of defense for our body, they are there to protect the interface between our inside and our outside environment, and we totally kill off that protection when we use a product made with bee's wax.

So you see, we need to understand *how* this body works and *what* life is, so we can give this body, this life, all the help we can to be healthy and beautiful. We can only do that by putting in and on our skin the compounds that enhance, feed, and promote life, physically as well as electrically. So anything we put on and into this body has to have the correct energy fields, the vibrational symphony of the impulses of life. And that means we should eat live, fresh food -- the way nature made it -- and very little food that is in a packet or that is processed. Drink the purest water possible -- never city tap water, as that is totally dead from chlorine and other chemicals. Put on our skin that which is not distorted, manufactured, processed, or preserved to the point that there is no life in it, and *never* use chemical-based skin creams or lotions.

"Sounds complicated," you say.

No, not really. Think about what was said earlier. If something does not decay (start to break down or rot) in a week at room temperature, then it is *not* food, you will get next to nothing from it, nor will it do your skin any good. Does your skin cream start to go rotten out of the tube in a week? Hell no. It will still look okay in 10 years.

If you still desire to use some good, high grade, natural oils on your skin, use them very sparingly, spread the oils very thin, and massage in well so that the critters can still get their oxygen and stay alive. Never forget: This life, this body, your skin, all of it, critters and all, inside and out, is and are living, breathing, biological life forms. If you disrupt or kill any of it in some way, then you -- this thing you think is you -- will not be, cannot be, healthy. And it's only a healthy cell that gives us beautiful skin and a healthy body.

7. CREATING OUR DISEASE

"And that's not all!"

As the now-famous saying screams from our TVs. No indeed, that is not all. Since our skin is, as you now know, an absorbable organ, then what we put on our skin can, and very often does, penetrate through to our blood. That is why, good people, hormonal creams and nicotine patches work. Chemicals and lots of other compounds can and do enter our blood through our skin. In fact, our skin can be classed in some ways as more absorbable that our stomach. I have clients who can eat small amounts of a lemon with no problems, but put just the smallest drop of lemon juice on their skin, and their body goes into shock. We all know about the effects on our skin and body of stinging nettle, don't we? So yes; the skin is very reactive, and that reactivity affects every other cell in our body as well. However, petrochemical compounds (and mineral oil is one) get through to our blood lickety-split (fast as).

It's quite frightening to think that the average woman applies something like 80 million non-life-giving chemical molecules a day to her blood with her daily skin care regime. That's about two and a half pounds of death going into her blood stream every year. And you wonder why I have been screaming for years for woman to STOP using chemical skin creams.

But before we talk about the electrical -- the energy -- damage we do to our body's energy system, I will give a short rundown of the physical damage that can transpire with this chemical loading for those who have not read my other books.

When the chemical bits get into your blood, your body has no idea what they are; they cannot be part of the life-giving process, but they also cannot stay in your blood, as your blood has a very defined set of parameters. And non-life-giving, man-made chemicals are not part of that. So the body has to put these chemicals somewhere. In a young girl, these chemicals get pushed to the outer layers of fatty tissue just under the skin, out of harm's way from the life support systems. It is this chemical build up in the inner layers of the skin that is the cause of skin cancer, NOT THE SUN. But that's another book all on its own.

However, a small side note: If you think about it, we humans would be long wiped out if sun on skin caused cancer. Also, every New Zealand farmer would be riddled with skin cancer, as they get sun on their faces and arms every day of their lives. So why do we all get told today to keep out of the sun and plaster sun block on our bodies? Well maybe because sun on skin produces the most *anti-cancer* compound known: Vitamin D$_3$. And keeping us *out* of the sun will increase the profits of the cancer industry. Another thing: In my mother's day, all the birthing homes had a sun room, and all the mothers and babies had to spend time in there to get sun on themselves and their babies (the old mid-wives knew a thing or two). One of the most maddening practices for me today is to see young mothers walking around with their babies all covered up. I feel like telling (and sometimes do) the young mums to take off the covering and let the baby's skin get some sun. In fact, sun on skin is one of the healthiest things we can do for ourselves and our babies. There are many scientific papers that show that those who sun-bathe, have far less cancer and live longer than those who don't. Once again: God (nature) did not get it wrong. We evolved in the sun. Sun gives life; it does not take life away.

Skin cancer is only a small part of the problem; there is much more damage being done -- life-destroying damage -- from this toxic chemical infusion through your skin. Bear with me now, and follow my train of thought, as this is profound stuff.

The chemicals from the young girls' skin creams, lotions, sun blocks, sun screens, even the baby creams her mother put on her skin as a baby (and Vaseline and mineral oils are petrochemicals), are all now stored in the fatty tissue just under the skin. Hold on to that.

When the young girl grows up and starts a family, her fetus gets its first trimester nourishment, its life giving food if you like, from the essential fatty acid reserves from the mother, not from the food the mother eats at the time.

All fetuses are female at the start of life (yes guys, we all start out as female, hormonally that is, even if we have the male chromosome coded into our little developing bodies).

It takes a series of hormonal triggers to go off in that first trimester to change a developing body containing the male chromosome, to that of a male hormonal profile. Yes, hormonally we change from female to male in that time.

Now (and this is where and how things go haywire), as the fetus is getting its nourishment from the very parts of the mother's body that also happens to be the chemical waste dump from her chemical skin products, the nourishment being pumped into the baby is loaded with these chemicals. Millions and millions of molecules of the stuff.

It is a known fact that petrochemical compounds are, or act as, hormonal mimics; that is, the body thinks that it is a hormone of some kind and this confusion can, and often does, stop or at least disrupt the hormonal changes that are meant to take place. So the boy baby grows with male chromosomes and male body parts but with varying levels of a *female* hormonal profile. Now you can see why I talked about the low sperm count in the young boys earlier. But that's not all: A male body with too many female hormones, will not only have a lower sperm count, suffer penile erectile issues, and in some cases suffer from short penis syndrome, but can also, as the ratio of female hormones goes up, have more and more female tendencies. He will feel and act female, display female temperament, and with a high enough female hormonal profile, will in essence *be* a female in a man's body. We call that *gay*, or as we call it in science, *cross-gender*. All our sexual tendencies, all our sexual desires, our thought processes, our behavior patterns, our likes and dislikes, are *hormonally* driven. We *are* what our *hormones* are.

Being gay is not a choice; it is *hormonally* driven. And it was the chemical loading from our mothers that triggered the whole hormonal-blocking phenomenon. It is not my belief. It is not what I *think* happens; this is a scientific fact. The hormonal changes only take place in the first trimester, and the only way the fetus can get the chemicals at that time is from the mother's essential fatty reserves, which happen to be the body's chemical storage dump in young girls. And the biggest way (really one of the only ways) that the girls had this chemical loading in their fatty tissue, was from the chemical-infused creams and lotions that were applied to their skin. An interesting side note: The biggest users of Viagra are not the 60 to 70 year-olds. It's not even the 50 to 60 year-olds; it's the 30 to 40 year-olds. I rest my case. We are living in a time of mass de-malenation of our males all caused by the beauty industry and its chemical-based skin products.

Yes, the female fetus can get hormonally screwed as

well. However, nowhere near as much as the male fetus, because there is not as much electrical triggering involved, as they do not have to change their hormonal profile in the first trimester; thus, less chance for a mishap.

Another point: We have all heard about some bad side effects of immunization, and that's a good debate. There is even a new movie on that issue. But when I look at the destruction of all health, from hormonal chaos, to emotional swings, to cross-gender issues, low sperm count, toxic bodies, obesity, arthritis, diabetes, and the explosion in women's *cancer,* and all the other degenerative diseases, there is NO doubt in my mind, that the biggest contributor, by far, is the cosmetics industry and their *chemical-based* skin creams and lotions. Our over-indulgence in refined carbs, grain, sugar and artificial sweeteners, soy, and other crap, non-food is a close second. (And oh, by the way; when you microwave anything you instantly turn every molecule in the food into a carcinogen. The electrical field of the food is totally destroyed).

I often ask: "So where is the movie about the chemical cosmetic industry?" The chemical-based cosmetic industry causes far more disease and destruction, to a larger percentage of the population, than anything else.

But all this is not new. We agriculturalists have known this since the 1970s, and numerous scientists have produced many papers on the subject; however, one of the best arguments on this subject is a book titled, *Our Stolen Future*, by Theo Colborn, Dianne Dumanoski and

John Peterson Myers. Read that book, and then try to tell me I do not know what I am talking about. I have been telling every female client of mine for over 30 years to stop using any product on her skin with chemicals in it. In fact, I will not work with any breast cancer client unless she agrees to never use chemical-based skin products.

It was this knowledge -- this destruction of our breeding capacity, this disease-causing (breast cancer) and cross-gender explosion relating to chemical skin creams and lotions -- that was the motivation for me to change my life nine or ten years ago. I embarked on a journey to find the most powerful and life-giving natural food and figure out how to make the world's first biologically-alive, life-giving, chemical-free skin cream with it.

That journey provided me with the science and the reasons I needed to form our company: The Human Experience, which now has a line of chemical-free skin care products. Thus far, nine of them are colostrum-based creams, and two are amazing, botanical essential-oil-based lotions which also contain colostrum oil. Each one is a world first. Our brand is called *theCream*. We do not manufacture our skin creams and lotions; we *craft* them. We do not use big automated machines, but rather, each and every batch is crafted by hand, by real people. We only use the best ingredients: the best colostrum and the best botanical oils. Every ingredient has its electrical field looked at and approved by me. We hand batch every run to ensure the vibrational field in the finished product is intact, and that it has the symphony of life within its field. We only use full-spectrum lighting in our plant, and all our mixers rotate in a clockwise direction (I could write another book on these two issues, but suffice to say, all things get affected by light (energy), just ask any indoor grower of plants, and all molecules electrical fields get affected by rotation. We use all known science to craft the most electrically (energy) perfect products). I know of no other skin care company that has incorporated the level of attention to detail and the understanding of the energy fields into the crafting of its products -- than we do.

Also ladies, when you use a water-based chemical skin cream, you are actually paying for 60-80% water, as water is the first ingredient. Therefore, if you paid $20 for that skin cream, you are paying a $1 for each percentage of so-called chemical active (the 20% that's left), after the water that does nothing, is taken out of the equation. However, when you buy a skin cream that has as its first ingredient a powerful active, with no added water, as in our colostrum cream, and even if it costs $70, you are actually only paying 70 cents per active ingredient, because the whole tube is made of actives (100% divided by $70 is 70 cents). Thus it's 30% cheaper to use than your chemical based $20 cream. Then due to its energetic and life-giving function on the skin, you only need to use half as much is you would normally use, thus the cost comes down to 70% less than a water-based, chemical skin cream. Think about this next time you are about to spend your hard earned dollars.

This life we live is our *only human experience,* and if we keep heading down our current path, that human experience will soon be impossible. We are already the most diseased, the most toxic, the lowest sperm count, the lowest life-energy, and the most hormonally-screwed group of people -- right here, right now -- to ever have a human experience. If we do not wake up and see, and then change, the reality of our chemically-toxic bodies and our world, we are surely doomed.

Okay, so far, we have covered the way our bodies store the non-life-giving and chemical molecules when we are young; now we will look at what the body does with these chemicals when we get older.

As women mature, their breasts develop and grow. Now, the breast is largely made up of fatty tissue, which now becomes the perfect store house for any non-life-giving compounds and chemicals. As you women (and more and more men) keep putting on your chemical-based creams and lotions, in your genetically-driven urge to look young and beautiful, these chemicals get through to your blood; the lymphatic system filters these out and creates a pathway and deposits the chemical molecules and other garbage, in a nice little "jail" in the breast tissue, out away from the life support organs inside your body. As you know, molecules are very small bits of stuff, so it takes many millions of them, over many years, before you become aware of this chemical 'jail'. This first shows up as a small lump, and it is only then that you might look a bit deeper into what is going on; however, by then the chemicals have, by and large, caused enough of an electrical system stress that some cells could well have started to malfunction into what we call cancer.

Good people, *you do not catch* cancer. It is *caused*. You cannot cure something that is caused. One can only stop the cause and then attempt to treat the damaged cells to bring them back into homeostasis, or what we call health. Most of us think of cancer as something going wrong, a sickness of some cells. But a cancerous cell is not sick in the way we normally understand *sickness*; rather, it is a cell that has lost its electrical feed to its instruction book -- its energy connection with its genetic code -- and so it is off and running at full speed, not knowing where to or why. It has lost its ability to regulate -- limit or govern -- its protein intake, so it grabs as much as it can and thus grows at a speed faster than the cells around it. It is so hungry, it devours anything and everything in its path. A sick, weak cell it is not; it's a fully-loaded runaway eighteen wheeler, without a driver, with its throttle jammed wide open gaining speed, going down a big hill. Trouble is, it's about as destructive as that out-of-control eighteen wheeler as well, and the path that it is destroying is *you*.

Another misconception: We do not actually die of or from cancer. As I said, a cancer cell is not a sick, low-energy cell; it is a full-on power house of a cell. However, it is so destructive in its overpowering ability that it consumes everything in its path. So eventually there are not enough correctly-functioning cells in the organ that the cancer cells are operating in to keep the organ working. You die of organ failure.

That's why chemotherapy drugs have such an abysmal success rate with such debilitating side effects (The *NCI Journal* 87:10, in an article by John Diamond, M.D. states: "In a study of over 10,000 patients, those who underwent chemo were 14 times more likely to develop leukemia and 6 times more likely to develop cancers of the bones, joints, and soft tissues than those patients who did not undergo chemotherapy"). The drugs are trying to kill the cancer cells. Trouble is, the cancer cells are much stronger than your good cells, so to knock out the cancer cells, you all but kill the good cells. To my way of thinking, trying to kill a very strong cell, to the detriment of all the other cells in the body is asinine. Remember: The only way to stop something happening is to figure out *how* it happened in the first place. Then and only then can you stop it happening.

So what caused the cell to lose its electrical connection to its instruction book in the first place? A toxic chemical molecule in most cases, but also an impact or perhaps other issues that shocked or lowered the energy feed to the cell's DNA. Pain is really just a low-energy alarm. That's why if you hit yourself, the energy gets dissipated from the cells and "on" goes the alarm, which is your pain.

However, in nearly all breast cancer, the cause is that the energy field around a chemical molecule is so powerful, so out-of-phase with the symphony of life, the chemicals field overpowered or short circuited the energy field of the breast cell. Thus, the breast cell lost its electrical feed to its instruction book -- its genetic code -- and off it went in a feeding and growing frenzy not knowing what it was meant to do. So it did nothing for the body, but it did everything for itself, and that was to grow very fast and overpower everything around it. Quite simple really. That's why I call cancer *chemical toxicity*. If the chemical was not there, the cells would not have their energy fields distorted, would not have lost their energy connection to their DNA, and thus would not have gone haywire and out of control. Cancer is not a sickness; it's an electrical malfunction, a short circuit if you like, that is caused by a stronger, or out-of-phase *unnatural* electrical field, and the electrical fields of chemicals are just that.

Okay, so let's back up a bit, shall we? If the girl did not get chemical-based creams or mineral oils on her skin as a baby, if she did not use her mother's chemical-based skin creams and chemical sun screens and sun blocks as a teenager, if she did not buy her own chemical-based skin creams as a young woman, then the fatty tissue layer under her skin would not be full of chemicals. Therefore, when she got pregnant no chemicals would have gotten to her fetus, and there would have been no chance that any chemical's energy construct would have overpowered the very delicate energy impulses that were meant to trigger the hormonal changes in her boy fetus. Thus, the fetus would have grown with its correct hormonal profile. Girls would grow up to be women, and boys would become men.

Then, if the young woman did not continue to use

chemical-based skin and sun products into her adult life, her breasts would not have been used as convenient chemical waste dumps; therefore, there would not have been an *unnatural* chemical energy field to overpower the breast cell's energy field, so the breast cells would not have lost their energy connection to their DNA, and thus would not have run-amok. No -- or very little -- breast cancer. Period.

I won't go into the stupidity of how the medical profession tries to treat cancer. Suffice to ask: Why don't we just inject a few penny's-worth of cannabis oil directly into the out-of-control cancer cells and let nature's strong energy field bring it back under control? Why don't we fire a shot of radio frequency energy, with the pin-point accuracy of a machine worth a few hundred dollars, into the cancer cells to give them a taste of what they are doing to other cells and knock their energy field for six? Why don't we go to a knowledgeable energy healer and pay him or her a few hundred dollars at the first sign of cancer, and get the cells rewired and electrically reformatted so they can once again receive their electrical feed from their DNA code?

Why don't we know about these and hundreds of other non-invasive natural health treatments? Like why is it not common knowledge that by taking the right amount of Selenium supplements, we could lower all cancers by about 70%? Us farmers always feed our animals minerals to keep them at peak health, so why aren't we humans taking minerals every day? By taking minerals, which become mineral salts in our body, we fortify the electrical processes in our body, as electrical current travels better in a saline solution. That is why we get a saline drip when we get rushed into the emergency room. Or give children electrolytes when they are sick. Get it? It's all about energy and the electrical process that *is* life.

Then again, why do we use hundreds of thousands of dollars-worth of even more toxic chemicals (drugs) called chemotherapy and more hundreds of thousands of dollars in toxic radiation treatments that we know after decades of use, don't really work? Oh yes, how silly of me; it's called *money*.

One last side note: The three leading causes of death in the USA in descending order are: Heart disease (which you do not *'catch'*), cancer (which you do not *catch*), and Medical Errors (mistakes by medical professionals). Medical mistakes, as reported by Johns Hopkins Medicine researchers, include incorrect diagnoses, preventable complications, and medication mix-ups (including poisonous overdoses; yes, death by man-made chemicals, people). The number of deaths, in the USA, by medical mistakes is reported to be 250,000 per year. I have seen other reports that state the real number is as high as 400,000. Think about that: In five or so years, our so called "health" system kills more people *by mistakes* than the U.S. military has lost in all overseas wars they've engaged in.

Another interesting point I have always thought about: There are 38,000 road deaths per year in the USA. And all these deaths are due to 'mistakes' in one way or another. We spend hundreds of millions in policing our roads, investigating the mistakes (accidents), and prosecuting millions. We are always told the traffic police, speed limits, and driving citations (fines) are in place to reduce the death toll. Strange that. If it was *really* about preventing deaths, one would think that all those police officers and prosecutors would be assigned to the hospitals, because *that* is where most of the deaths due to mistakes happen. Maybe, just maybe, it's not about death, but about easy revenue -- as I said above; it's called money. The sad part of all this BS, is that we the people, allow all this to take place: We keep electing, year after year, the very people who tell us the lies and take our money under false pretenses. It's also interesting to note that Germany, which has the lowest number of roads with speed limits, gives out the lowest number of traffic tickets and, has the lowest death rate per mile driven in the western world. Just had to point that out. Now back to where we were.

Over the last three decades of my work, I have seen many thousands of women and their kids. I have seen most every problem and issue that is inflicted upon our modern world and its people. However, by far the most devastating cause of most of their health issues, is their lack of knowledge about *how* health problems happen. We are so tied up with naming disease, we forget that 90% of what ails us is caused by our ignorance, our lack of knowing *how* it happened. And of course, most of our so-called diseases are degenerative diseases, and we do not *catch* those. They are self-inflicted.

I could have written another 20,000 words, but that is not the point. What I set out to do is to show you, the reader, that your body is much more, way more, than you have ever realized. Also, all my experience has given this old brain of mine a darn good insight into the biggest problems and the root of some of our most pressing health issues. There is no doubt in my mind, when I take everything into account, that the last 50 years or so of chemical "stuff" we have plastered on our skin has caused more real long term harm to us, to our children, and even to their children than all the other potential dangers we confront in life.

We are told every day how bad for our health smoking is, but listen up: One month of the average Western woman's skin care regime is more toxic, more disease-causing to you and your children than is 10 years of heavy smoking. Breathe that in (pun intended). One in three smokers do not die from smoking; however, one in three of you ladies have or will have some form of serious disease (mainly breast cancer) in the next 20 years if we keep going the way we are heading. The point is that most, if not all, of your health challenges (and this is my humble opinion) will be triggered by chemicals and the devastating electrical damage they do to your systems. And the biggest and most perfect way the chemicals get into your body is through your skin: Your *chemical skin creams* are by far the most destructive, abusive, and disease-causing products that you will inflict on yourself in your life.

This is why I have dedicated my life to looking into,

changing, and informing you all about this devastation.

I have put everything I have into formulating a safe, natural, life-giving skin care line because I could not live with myself if, knowing what I know, I did nothing. Colostrum is *God's* (nature's) most powerful life-giving food, and that's what my product line, *theCream*, is made from.

However, you have many new ideas to think about: The food you put in your body, your hormones, your skin, nearly every system gets knocked for six with refined carbs, soy, microwaves, too much sugars, etc. So hopefully, as now you have read my words, you, that wonderful, amazing, alive, life-giving woman can take some of your power back, make some better choices, and live and BE that amazing, loving, empowered, vibrant goddess you came to experience in this life.

I just hope I have been able to give you all something to hold on to. Take it as yours; it's your life, but even more than that: It is *you*. My only wish is for all of you to be happy, be at peace inside, be healthy, a little crazy, but most of all, be *all* of you. And know that you are beautiful.

We came to live this life full of love, joy, happiness with vibrant health and to look and feel great well into our old age. We came to dance, be a little crazy, and live every moment to its fullness.

Denie Hiestand

EPILOGUE

There is no freedom, there cannot be democracy and there is no humanity, when the masses are living a delusional life based on an illusion created by the few.

America's so-called democracy, the cosmetic industry, and big pharma are perfect bedfellows; they have all endeavored to cover up any truth and fool the very people who gave them their trust and wealth.

From an abundance of life, comes an abundance of free thought. From an abundance of free thought, comes the power to change our world and to free ourselves from the shackles of illusion.

Denie Hiestand

.

ABOUT THE AUTHOR

Denie Hiestand, originally from New Zealand, is now based in Las Vegas, Nevada. He is a world-renowned Natural Health Consultant, author, seminar presenter and creator of healthy skin care products. His other books include: *Electrical Nutrition*, *Journey to Truth* (also made into an award winning documentary film, *One Man's Journey to Truth,* by Chesapeake Films) and *A Little Book of Wisdom*. For more information please visit: www.theCream.com

Made in the
USA
Lexington, KY